# GARLIC

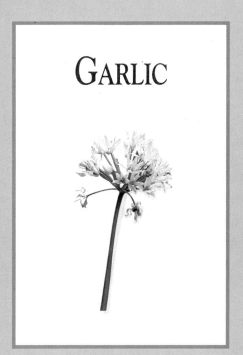

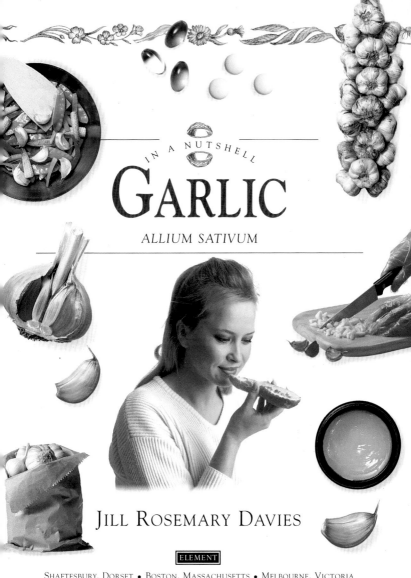

# IN A NUTSHELL

# GARLIC

*ALLIUM SATIVUM*

# JILL ROSEMARY DAVIES

ELEMENT

SHAFTESBURY, DORSET • BOSTON, MASSACHUSETTS • MELBOURNE, VICTORIA

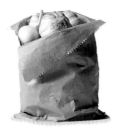

© Element Books Limited 2000

First published in Great Britain in 2000 by
ELEMENT BOOKS LIMITED
Shaftesbury, Dorset SP7 8BP

Published in the USA in 2000 by
ELEMENT BOOKS INC.
160 North Washington Street,
Boston MA 02114

Published in Australia in 2000 by
ELEMENT BOOKS LIMITED
and distributed by Penguin Australia Ltd
487 Maroondah Highway,
Ringwood, Victoria 3134

NOTE FROM THE PUBLISHER
Any information given in this book is not
intended to be taken as a replacement for
medical advice. Any person with a condition
requiring medical attention should consult
a qualified practitioner or therapist.
For growing and harvesting, calendar
information applies only to the northern
hemisphere (US zones 5–9).

Jill Rosemary Davies has asserted her right
under the Copyright, Designs, and Patents
Act, 1988, to be identified as Author of
this work.

Designed and created with
The Bridgewater Book Company Ltd.

ELEMENT BOOKS LIMITED
Managing Editor Miranda Spicer
Senior Commissioning Editor Caro Ness
Project Editor Kate John
Group Production Director Clare Armstrong
Production Manager Stephanie Raggett
Production Controller Claire Legg

THE BRIDGEWATER BOOK COMPANY
Art Director Rebecca Willis
Designer Jane Lanaway
Project Editor Lorraine Turner
Editorial Director Fiona Biggs
DTP Designer Chris Lanaway
Picture Research Lynda Marshall
Photography Guy Ryecart
Illustrations Michael Courtney

Printed and bound in Portugal by
Printer Portuguesa.

Cataloging in Publication data is
available from the Library of Congress

Cataloguing in Publication data is
available from the British Library

ISBN 1 86204 559 3

The publishers wish to thank the
following for the use of pictures:
A–Z Botanical Collection: pp.2, 6r, 7, 8,
9t, 13t, 13bl.
Bridgeman Art Library: pp.10b,
British Museum, London; 55, Musée
D'Orsay, Paris.
E. T. Archive: p.11t.
Garden Picture Library: pp.10t, 23, 25.
Image Bank: pp.13br, 17, 21t, 31, 43, 53b.
Science Photo Library: p.14b.
The Dr. Christopher family, Utah: p.45.

Special thanks go to:
Kay Macmullan for arranging
photography

# Contents

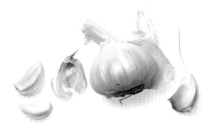

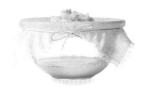

# Introduction

*WELL KNOWN FOR ITS CULINARY USES, Garlic is also an outstanding medicinal herb. Its antibiotic properties make it useful for fighting a wide range of infections in both humans and animals, protecting and prolonging life for all concerned.*

Garlic, which is widely cultivated commercially, may grow to be 1–3ft (30–90cm) tall. The bulb below ground is the main part of the plant to be used medicinally and is divided into segments called cloves. Each bulb contains between 6 and 12 cloves, which often vary tremendously in size depending on the soil conditions.

## DEFINITION

Botanical family: *Liliaceae* (though it is sometimes assigned to *Alliaceae*).
Species: *Allium sativum* is the Garlic species that is most frequently used medicinally and, unless otherwise stated, is the species referred to in this book. There are 500 other members of the Allium family, including leeks, onions, chives, and shallots, as well as different types of garlic suitable for medicinal use in a similar manner to *A. sativum*.

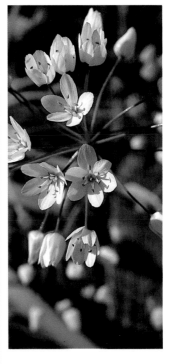

ABOVE **Ramsons (A. ursinum)** *produces delicate white flowers in the summer.*

An erect stem grows from the Garlic bulb to form an umbrella-shaped arrangement of flowers clustered together, with linear leaves growing from the base of the stem. The flower cluster, swathed in a papery sheath, varies in color from purplish white to pale pink or a reddish white, according to the species, soil, and chemical influences. The aromatic, attractive flowers have many small bulbils in between them. Black seeds, which form after flowering has finished (between July and September), ripen in wild Garlic species, but will not do so in cultivated varieties.

Garlic's familiar smell derives from its sulfur-containing constituents, which also give the herb its medicinal properties. If you crush a clove, allicin is released, which converts to odorous diallyl disulfite.

A traditional antidote to the lingering smell of Garlic is to chew a sprig of parsley.

There are many closely related species of Garlic. In Britain these include wild Field Garlic (*Allium oleraceum*), which is a common sight in the early summer and

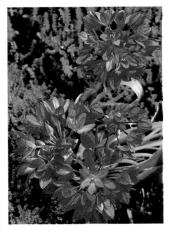

ABOVE *Some species of Garlic, such as* A. oreophilum *pictured here, produce colorful, pink flowers.*

grows in damp hedgerows and along riverbanks. It has small but strong-smelling bulbs.

Ramsons (*A. ursinum*) is another common *Allium* species. It has very broad leaves that make it an excellent, pungent addition to a salad. Ramsons has many of the same medicinal uses as Garlic and a long history as a healing herb, as this ancient Old English rhyme attests:

*Eat Leeks in Lide and*
*Ramsons in May*
*And all the year after*
*physicians may play!*

# Exploring Garlic

GARLIC HAS A HISTORY OF RECORDED USE *stretching back about 5,000 years. Some believe it originated in Central Asia, while others think it came from the Kirgiz desert in Western Siberia. Today it is widely cultivated around the world.*

## WHERE TO FIND GARLIC

Both wild and cultivated varieties of Garlic grow all over the globe. The herb can be found growing in Asia, Egypt, Pakistan, China, Russia, and the United States, and in Mediterranean regions of Europe, for example, in Greece, Italy, Spain, and France.

Field Garlic (*A. oleraceum*) can be found growing wild in parts of Britain, notably in Yorkshire and Derbyshire, but Ramsons (*A. ursinum*) is the most common

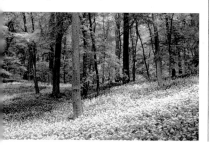

type of wild Garlic in Britain. It grows on rich, loamy, mildly acidic soil and is self-pollinated. Unlike Garlic, Ramsons is used mainly for its leaves.

In the United States, Field Garlic (*A. vineale*), known as Crow Garlic in Britain, can be found in the fields of Massachusetts, Michigan, and New York State. It has attractive pink and white flowers and reaches a height of 1–3ft (30–90cm) depending on the soil. A similar looking type of wild Garlic (*A. canadense*) grows in meadows in Minnesota and Wisconsin, as well as in southern Ontario and Quebec in Canada. It has fewer flowers than Field Garlic and only grows to 1–1½ft (30–45cm) in height.

LEFT **Carpets of white Ramsons in British woodlands are a breathtaking sight in the spring.**

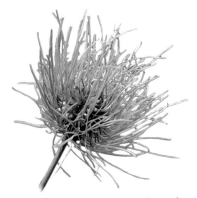

## COMMERCIAL GROWERS

Two countries produce the bulk of commercially grown Garlic, namely the United States and China. Other countries also produce large amounts, but primarily for their own needs with only a small quantity reserved for export.

## SOIL REQUIREMENTS

Although Garlic will grow almost anywhere, it thrives best in well-drained soil, preferably sandy or silty loam that is rich in organic matter. Ideally the pH should be neutral or slightly acid. This type of soil

is particularly suitable because it enables Garlic to establish a good root system, producing roots that can grow down for 2–3ft (60–90cm) and draw up plenty of moisture and nutrients. These nutrients are invaluable to the plant: they ensure that Garlic is rich in vital vitamins, minerals, and other important plant chemical constituents.

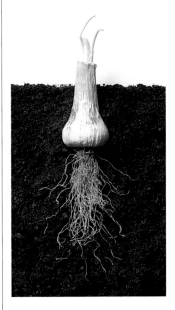

ABOVE *Garlic owes its rich
mineral content to an efficient
root system that reaches deep
down into the soil.*

# A history of healing

PROBABLY ONE OF THE OLDEST "cure-alls" in the world, Garlic was used by ancient cultures in many of the same ways as it is used today, to combat coughs, colds, and a host of other infections.

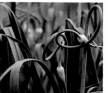

LEFT *The word "Garlic" means "spear plant." This species is* A. sativum.

## NAMES AND FOLKLORE

One of Garlic's common names is Poor Man's Treacle. "Treacle" derives from the Chaucerian word *theriac*, meaning "heal-all" –"poor man's heal-all" sums up Garlic's cheap, all-round healing properties.

The Anglo Saxons called the plant *garlac* or *garleac*, based on a visual description of the leaves: *gar* means "spear" or "lance" and *lac* means "plant"; *leac* means "potherb." Ajoene, one of Garlic's chemicals, takes its name from the Spanish for Garlic, *ajo*.

## TRADITIONAL USES

Garlic has a long history of medicinal use. Archeologists have found evidence of the herb in Egyptian tombs dating back to 3750BCE, and slaves in Egypt were given Garlic as part of their daily food ration. Garlic is not, however, mentioned in the records of Chinese medicine until 500CE.

BELOW *Slaves building the Great Pyramid were given Garlic to keep up their strength.*

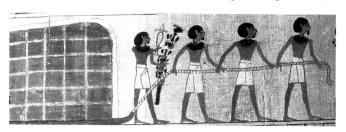

The ancient Greek scholar and herbalist Pliny listed 62 medicinal uses for Garlic, and Aristotle recommended it as a treatment for rabies. Other historical uses for Garlic include the treatment of leprosy, scorpion bites, scrofulous sores, smallpox, and anthrax.

The Vikings and Phoenicians put Garlic in their seachests before starting long voyages, and in Romany lore it is one of the five healing foods (the others are onion, lemon, chili, and honey).

Garlic's anti-infective properties have long been put to good use. In medieval times, the famous French "Four Thieves' Mixture," which contained Garlic, is said to have enabled grave robbers to plunder graves without contracting the plague. In World War I, sphagnum moss, which has antimicrobial properties, was soaked in diluted Garlic juice and bandaged onto wounds to help control infection and assist healing. During World War II, the Russians practiced the same methods. Furthermore, syrup of Garlic was, for many centuries, used to treat respiratory diseases such as

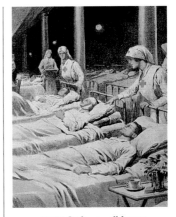

ABOVE *Garlic, a well-known antibiotic, was used to treat wounds during World War I.*

bronchitis, colds, asthma, coughs, tuberculosis, and whooping cough.

Garlic is a traditional worming remedy. In India and the West it is added to milk and drunk to expel intestinal worms. In India, Garlic has been used in a variety of other ways, in particular to treat diabetes.

In the past, Garlic was used to treat skin disorders such as acne, as well as high blood pressure, low blood pressure, and a range of heart complaints including angina. Garlic has also been a circulatory remedy since Roman times.

# Anatomy of Garlic

THE GARLIC BULB *is used medicinally. Other parts of the plant have the same constituents, but to a lesser degree. Generally the leaves, flowers, and stems are not used medicinally, although they are a healing food.*

## BULBS

Garlic bulbs can vary tremendously in size and color, according to their variety and the soil in which they have been grown. The *Allium sativum* bulb, when fresh, is held together by several layers of whitish to pinkish purple skin (the color is dependent on the species). Inside this skin lie a number of grouped bulblets, or cloves, of varying sizes and shapes. These plump and generally half-moon-shaped cloves are enclosed in membranous white coverings. After being peeled for consumption, the cloves inside are smooth and pearly-white in color.

RIGHT *Garlic bulbs are composed of 6 to 12 segments, known as cloves.*

## Chemical constituents

Garlic's main active constituent is alliin, which is contained in its volatile oil. When crushed, alliin converts to allicin. Allicin and other constituents of the oil are antiseptic. Other constituents include minerals such as zinc, calcium, iron, magnesium, potassium, and trace minerals; vitamins (mainly A, B, C, and E); and enzymes, carbohydrates, essential oils, fatty acids, sterols, flavonoids, nucleosides, anthocyanins, and more than 200 other sulfur compounds. Garlic also contains 17 amino acids, which include lysine, arginine, and cysteine.

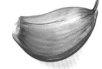

## STEMS AND LEAVES

Similar in appearance to grass, the leaves of Garlic are long, narrow, and flattened. The tops of the leaves form a point, and at their base they wrap around the stem until one side of the leaf meets the other. Garlic stems and leaves have some of the same constituents as the bulb, and may be eaten as a healing food.

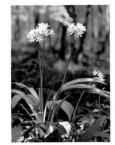

ABOVE *A. ursinum leaves fan out from the base of the stem.*

## FLOWERS AND SEEDS

The flowers, which bloom in the summer, are located at the top of the stalk, which rises straight from the bulb. The flowers are grouped together in a spathe, which is a rounded, globular head with a translucent whitish-green cover that resembles a "pixie-hat." The delicate flowers come in a variety of white and cream shades, although occasionally they are lilac or pink. The flowers look pretty in salads and are a useful tonic food. Alternatively, they can be left to bloom and seed for decoration well into the fall, or can be dried for use in floral arrangements.

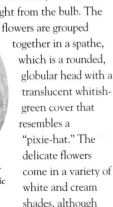

ABOVE *Like other species, Field Garlic flowers produce black seeds.*

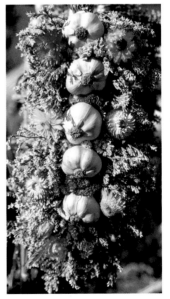

ABOVE *Decorative braided Garlic and flowers make an attractive display.*

# Garlic in action

GARLIC IS ONE OF THE *most popular and well-established healers in the herbal repertoire. In Germany, Garlic preparations outsell all other herbs, and so important is the plant that one pharmaceutical company even made a bid to patent some of its constituents. Among its many actions, Garlic reduces blood cholesterol, stabilizes blood-sugar levels, and is an important natural antibiotic. It also helps people with allergies by clearing allergens and heavy metals from the body.*

ABOVE
*Tablets contain synthesized form of Garlic's active constituents.*

## HOW GARLIC CAN HELP

Eating garlic regularly can help to ease circulatory and heart complaints, ranging from high or low blood pressure, to angina. Heart disease can arise for many different reasons, but one common cause is excessive amounts of cholesterol in the blood, which build up into plaque deposits that block the coronary arteries. These can cause angina, a severe pain that indicates the heart is not receiving sufficient blood.

Regular ingestion of Garlic can help to lower blood cholesterol levels significantly. This in turn can drastically reduce angina, and in some cases may even help to prevent heart attacks.

Garlic is able to improve the quality of the blood by raising the level of hemoglobin and the red blood cell count – this is very helpful for people with anemia (but see page 19).

BELOW *Laboratory tests show that Garlic helps to increase red blood cells.*

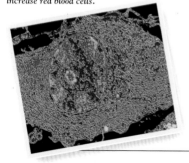

Statistics show that in countries where Garlic is eaten frequently, the immune systems of indigenous peoples are generally more active in fighting off cancer; in particular, fewer deaths from stomach cancer are recorded. Garlic appears to block the formation of cancer-causing compounds, preventing their ability to form tumors.

The Nobel Prizewinner Dr. Arthur Stoll proved that Garlic is an important antimicrobial agent. It can treat a variety of disorders from whooping cough and colds, to candida and salmonella infections, worm and parasitic infestations, dysentery, diarrhea, and constipation. Old remedies abound for using Garlic to treat respiratory problems varying from the common cold or sore throat, to emphysema, pneumonia, and tuberculosis. Particularly now that overuse of antibiotics is becoming increasingly common, Garlic is most useful as a natural antibiotic.

Garlic is helpful for diabetics too because it helps to stabilize blood-sugar levels and encourages the pancreas to produce insulin. It is also a fine

## GARLIC'S TONIC EFFECT

Reduces allergic reactions

Boosts resistance to coughs and colds

Protects against stomach cancer

Stabilizes blood-sugar levels

Aids recovery from diarrhea

Thins the blood, helping the circulation

ABOVE *Eating Garlic every day is excellent for good health and longevity.*

antiallergy food that helps to ease hay fever, asthma, allergic rhinitis, and food allergies.

Garlic seems to normalize the metabolism, and it also helps to detoxify the body's systems by binding with heavy metals and other harmful pollutants and destroying them.

# HOW GARLIC AFFECTS THE BODY

## Antibacterial remedy

Garlic is an antibiotic. It destroys a range of invasive microbes, including the bacteria that cause anthrax and tuberculosis. It also helps to fight infections of the digestive tract.

## Effective antiparasitic

An effective antiparasitic agent, Garlic helps to displace parasitic infestations such as *Giardia lamblia* and *Endameba histolytica*. These organisms are sensitive to the sulfur compounds (particularly allicin) in Garlic.

**GARLIC AND BODY SYSTEMS**

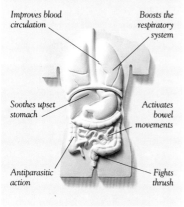

*Improves blood circulation*

*Boosts the respiratory system*

*Soothes upset stomach*

*Activates bowel movements*

*Antiparasitic action*

*Fights thrush*

## Blood improver

Some of Garlic's healing abilities are due to its fibrinolytic action, which increases the speed at which blood flows around the system, making it less likely to clot and resulting in faster circulation and better metabolism of oxygen. The compound in Garlic that achieves this is ajoene (see page 10).

## Immunity enhancer

Garlic has the ability to improve the number of "helper suppressor cells" and blood platelet count in the body. It also increases the levels of globulin (protein from which antibodies are made) in the blood and stimulates macrophage activity (scavenger cells that destroy bacteria).

## Antifungal agent

Partly as a result of its antioxidant properties, Garlic has effective antifungal properties. In the case of the candida fungus (which causes thrush), Garlic attaches itself to the fungus and destroys it.

LEFT *Garlic has a wide-ranging beneficial effect on the digestive and respiratory systems.*

## Digestive remedy

The healing compounds in Garlic can both soothe an upset stomach and activate bowel movements by encouraging peristalsis (the wave-like action of the gut that propels food through it). Garlic destroys a range of bacteria, viruses, and fungi infecting the gut and boosts levels of beneficial intestinal bacteria, making it a good remedy for all-round digestive health (but see page 19).

## Cancer preventive

Garlic inhibits the formation of nitrosamine (cancer-inducing compounds) by stopping nitrosamines, which are toxic chemicals found in food and the environment, from binding to healthy cells. Garlic also stimulates liver enzymes that are thought to be partly responsible for anticarcinogenic reactions.

## Heart health and blood pressure

Allicin (a sulfur compound) accelerates the liver's ability to break down lipids (fatty substances called cholesterol and triglycerides), which will otherwise build up on the inside of artery walls and result in heart

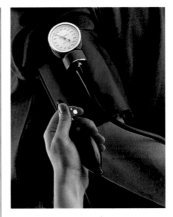

ABOVE *Garlic helps people with high blood pressure.*

disease. Garlic also contains anticoagulants that thin the blood and thereby reduce high blood pressure.

## Lung medicine

The sulfur compounds in Garlic work together to give the herb an expectorant action. Garlic reduces excessive mucus levels in the lungs, thus alleviating many bronchial disorders such as chronic catarrh and bronchitis.

## Degenerative diseases

Garlic has minerals and other constituents that act as antioxidants. They mop up free

17

radicals (harmful particles) that would otherwise damage the body. Thus Garlic helps prevent a range of degenerative diseases.

**Male sexual dysfunction**
According to Peter Josling, author of *The Complete Garlic Handbook* (see page 58), studies have shown that Garlic in certain forms can stimulate the production of nitric oxide synthase, which is primarily responsible for the mechanism of penile erection.

**Adrenal gland support**
Garlic increases production of monoamine oxidase (MAO) enzymes in the adrenal glands. MAO enzymes are responsible for breaking down and excreting adrenaline and other harmful chemicals from the blood. In this way, Garlic supports the systems and organs of the body, helping them to work efficiently.

## SUMMARY

Garlic should feature regularly on everyone's menu. It benefits a wide range of metabolic, cellular, and chemical processes in the body. In particular, it helps the digestive, circulatory, and immune systems to function at optimum level and it destroys harmful bacteria and free radicals. Truly, Garlic deserves its ancient reputation as a "cure-all."

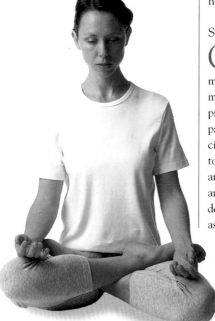

LEFT *Some devotees of yoga do not eat Garlic because its stimulating qualities disturb their concentration.*

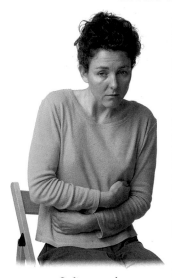

ABOVE *Garlic can soothe upset stomachs and encourage bowel movements by stimulating the action of the gut.*

## WHEN TO AVOID GARLIC

Most Europeans consume large amounts of Garlic without problem – it is a very safe herb. However, because of its stimulating qualities, practitioners of some forms of yoga are warned against eating it. Garlic can also occasionally damage blood cells and lead to anemia in some sensitive cases or where a person already suffers from ill-health. Bernard Jensen, the renowned American healer and herbalist, warns that eating more than one clove of raw Garlic a day on a long-term basis can irritate the bowel wall in some people. He also cautions that raw Garlic can cause heartburn, stomach ulcers, and wind.

People suffering from colitis may wish to try small amounts of Garlic first to make sure that it does not cause irritation.

When chopping very large quantities of Garlic, take care not to let it remain in contact with the skin for any length of time because it can burn. In small amounts, however, Garlic oil penetrating the skin will have a beneficial effect in the body.

BELOW *It is best to wear plastic gloves when handling large quantities of raw Garlic, because it can irritate the skin.*

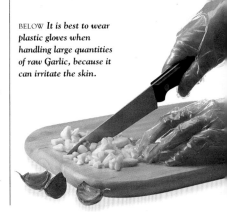

# Energy and emotion

WITH AN ANCIENT HISTORY *and remarkable properties, Garlic engenders a range of emotions and has an important place in folklore. Garlic is unparalleled in its strength, enabling the body to protect itself and taking over when the body is too weak to look after itself. It has long been believed that Garlic can ward off evil and in some cultures it has been adopted as a good-luck amulet.*

## TASTE

Hot, spicy Garlic has a central place at the heart of cuisines all over the world. Its powerful taste has always exerted an important influence on the emotions. In Chinese medicine, Garlic is viewed energetically as hot and spicy, with a particular affinity for the lungs, kidneys, spleen, stomach, and colon. It is a very stimulating, powerful, tonic food that benefits the whole digestive system from mouth to bowel.

LEFT *Who can resist the aroma of Garlic butter on freshly baked bread? Garlic's flavor can also be enhanced by roasting.*

## SMELL

Many people find the smell of Garlic unpleasant on the breath. Country, family, and social rituals must be taken into account when considering opinions on the odor of Garlic, but suffice to say that many Europeans are extremely relaxed and happy with its sulfurous smell.

The chemicals that give Garlic its smell also impart its healing properties, so "odor-free" products do not work as well as raw Garlic. It is possible that just inhaling Garlic's odor can help in the cure of some diseases, for example tuberculosis.

In traditional folklore, Garlic is held to protect against vampires, bats, and dark forces. It represents redemption from terrifying, otherworldly forces. Any truth in this reputation lies in the fact that Garlic helps to guard against physical, emotional, and mental disturbances. In some parts of the world, for example South America, Garlic is used to repel vampire bats, and it is fed to horses, cows, and other livestock to protect them against attacks from bats.

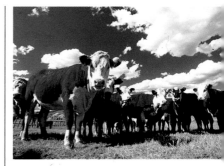

ABOVE *In some countries cows are fed Garlic to repel vampire bats, who dislike the taste.*

### CASE STUDY: ARTHRITIS

David Marshall, age 65, had very bad arthritis and suffered with pain in almost all his joints; in particular he had severe lower back pain. A friend suggested he take three lemons squeezed into spring water every morning and then consume a huge dose of raw garlic during the day. At first he ate only three cloves a day, then increased the dose to six cloves daily. He bravely mashed these into a little banana to help him consume them, half a clove at a sitting. After just one week his pains felt so much better that he was moving as he hadn't done for years. David soldiered on with this regime for a further month, before cutting back to a maintenance dose of three cloves a day.

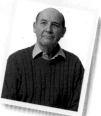

## FLOWER REMEDIES

Garlic flower essence is very purifying, and works on a subtle level. It may be taken orally or sprayed in the house. It imparts strength, is empowering, and gives confidence; it calms fears and anxieties, and prevents the individual from being overly influenced by outside forces, be they good, bad, or indifferent.

Garlic flower essence is said to have a special ability to keep away disturbing spirits who seek to integrate with the living – causing harm, unrest, or a reduction in vitality and energy. It fortifies the immune system and restores wholeness, strength, and harmony to mind and spirit.

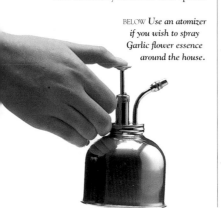

BELOW *Use an atomizer if you wish to spray Garlic flower essence around the house.*

## TO MAKE A FLOWER ESSENCE

### STANDARD QUANTITY

Approx 1½ cups (350ml) each of spring water and brandy, and 3–4 fresh Garlic flowers

1 *Submerge carefully chosen, freshly picked Garlic flowers in a glass bowl of shallow spring water. Cover the bowl with clean white cheesecloth.*

2 *Leave the bowl in sunshine for several hours or next to a window if indoors. Try to ensure that the flowers have at least three hours of continuous sun. If the flowers wilt sooner than this, they can be removed earlier.*

3 *After a few hours remove the flowers, using a twig to lift them out of the water.*

4 *Measure the remaining liquid and add an equal amount of brandy to preserve the essence. Pour into dark glass bottles and label these carefully.*

### Recommended dosage

✿ *Adults: 4 drops under the tongue 4 times daily, or every half hour in times of crisis. Children: over 12 years, adult dose; under 12 years, see page 43.*

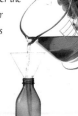

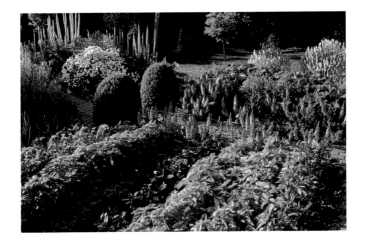

## PLANT SPIRIT ENERGIES

The spirit of the Garlic plant is different from the flower essence, which derives mostly from the flowering aspect of the plant. The whole spirit of the plant enables every part of it to share its energy with us.

Garlic is a supreme healer with high levels of purity; these qualities are reflected in its white color. Its ability to renew itself is arguably like any other plant that reappears from the earth each spring, but it has particularly strong antiaging abilities, which come from its antioxidant components.

ABOVE *The sulfurous compounds that Garlic exudes from its roots feed neighboring plants and protect them from infection.*

Even Garlic bulbs that are six months old have the ability to regenerate themselves.

Garlic is therefore an empowering plant for people, both mentally and physically. It is a plant that benefits not just humans and animals but also other plants; it is a wonderful companion plant and can help neighboring plants to resist disease and infection.

Take Garlic when a sense of wholeness, purity, and empowerment is needed.

# Growing, harvesting, and processing

GROWING YOUR OWN GARLIC *is easy and satisfying. It is a hardy plant, and whatever your soil type, given medium levels of fertility, you should be successful. Bernard Jensen, who is famed for his medicinal Garlic, insists that planting two days before a full moon will stimulate hardier, more bountiful growth. I have used moon cycles to grow Garlic and other plants and agree that it does make a difference.*

## GROWING GARLIC

As long as Garlic has a reasonable amount of sun, it will grow successfully in all temperate regions. Commercial growers do not always use *Allium sativum* but you should choose this because it is a good medicinal variety. The braided Garlic sold in many European markets often has a purple tinge to it, which may indicate growth hormones special to this species. It also has a very long, flowering stalk that is easy to braid. Some commercial growers for the food industry pick nonbolting or nonflowering types, and varieties grown in the United States include California Early, California Late, Roja, and Creole. There is also Elephant Garlic (*A. ampelprasum*), which is related to the leek; it produces enormous, easy-to-peel cloves.

BELOW **For home cultivation, choose** Allium sativum **cloves. Plant in fertile soil in a sunny spot.**

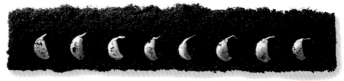

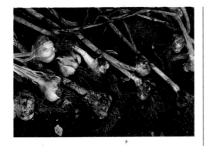

## GERMINATION

Choose large bulbs and divide them into cloves. Plant the cloves 2in (5cm) apart at a depth of 1–2in (2–5cm) with the pointed end upward. Plant in November, but in really cold areas wait until spring. Homegrown Garlic will produce the plumpest cloves if grown in medium, fertile soil with a range of nutrients including minerals and trace elements. Sandy or silty loam with a pH of acid to neutral often produces good results. Do not use chemical fertilizers – instead try well-rotted manure, leaves, or other organic fertilizers. Keep the area well weeded, ensuring you do not damage the surface roots.

RIGHT *Keep Garlic well weeded because weeds rob the soil of nutrients.*

LEFT *Growers of European Garlic keep the long, flowering stalk for braiding.*

Between March and May weeds are very active and can rob Garlic of local nutrients. Some natural mulch, such as hay or straw, will help to keep the moisture in. If it is very dry during May and June water the Garlic, allowing the cloves to plump up before harvesting. Some people suggest that if the soil has dried out, Garlic should be watered to a depth of 2ft (60cm) every 8 to 10 days. Stop watering four weeks before harvesting to allow the plants to dry out. Do not allow the plants to flower or seed because energy will be drawn away from the bulb.

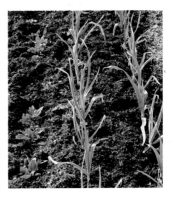

## HARVESTING

**Commercial** There are commercial Garlic farms worldwide, for instance in the United States, China, and Spain. Bulbs are uprooted by teams of laborers and spread out on slatted shelves in a cool, dry shed. Humidity levels are kept below 70 percent to ensure that bulbs are not infected with fungal spores or become moldy. Tops and roots are cut off within a few days and the extraneous mud is gently removed. Some Garlic stalks are left so that they can be braided.

**Homegrown** Harvesting usually takes place around the end of July for the main crop. However, in March and April you can crop the odd small bulb of Garlic, if required. The signal for harvesting Garlic is when the top

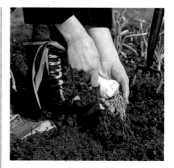

ABOVE *Holding the top, gently ease the Garlic bulb out of the ground.*

foliage starts to die down and shrivel. If it is a wet or damp summer, harvest quickly if you spot any fungal spores on the leaves. In very hot weather, the papery skin of the bulbs can split. This is not a problem, but an intact skin will protect the bulb and allow for better storage.

To harvest a bulb, hold the top then gently pull while easing the bulb free with a fork. Immediately chop off any withering or fungally infected leaves. This will prevent fungal infections or reduce their spread – surprisingly, Garlic can be particularly prone to them. Leave the roots and mud on; you can shorten the roots and knock off the dried mud later.

BELOW *After harvesting, Garlic bulbs are left to dry on wooden slatted shelves.*

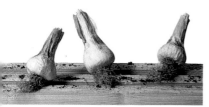

## PROCESSING

**Commercial** Growers must store their Garlic during final storage and shipment in the same careful conditions as before. A certain amount will be braided into ropes, known as "Ristras," while other bulbs will be carefully placed into wooden, slatted boxes. Each box of organically grown Garlic will be clearly labeled as such.

**Homegrown** Leave the Garlic stalks on because they are useful for hanging up the bulbs, but if fungal spores appear, you should chop off the stems immediately. Once the leaves have been removed, store the Garlic in a dry, cool area, preferably on slatted wooden shelves. Try not to knock the bulbs because they will bruise and consequently will not store well.

If they are stored properly, Garlic bulbs should last beautifully through the winter, and organically homegrown

ABOVE **Braiding Garlic is an attractive and practical way of storing the herb.**

bulbs always keep better than the commercial ones that have been grown with pesticide and chemical fertilizer. Remember that it is vital that the bulbs are stored somewhere that is well ventilated and well protected from frost.

For long-term storage, try putting Garlic into a paper bag and keeping it in the refrigerator. This will be especially useful during February and March when there is usually no outdoor-grown Garlic available, and will take you through to the new crop.

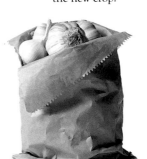

ABOVE **Garlic will keep for several months if stored in a paper bag in the refrigerator.**

# Preparations for internal use

GARLIC CLOVES CAN BE ENJOYED *cooked or eaten raw, and are delicious in salad dressings. As well as adding Garlic to most recipes, it is possible to take it in a variety of medicinal preparations, including tinctures, capsules, syrup, and fruit or vegetable juice.*

## GARLIC TINCTURE

Tinctures are one of the most convenient ways to take herbs, because as little as two or three drops can be the equivalent of drinking a whole cup of infusion. In the case of Garlic you would not readily wish to ingest the tincture on its own, because it is not

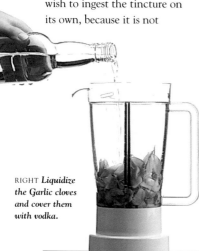

RIGHT *Liquidize the Garlic cloves and cover them with vodka.*

particularly palatable, but added to other herbs in a composite formula, or turned into a syrup, it is invaluable for treating a wide range of diseases.

Garlic tincture is made by soaking crudely chopped, unskinned cloves in alcohol to kill any germs and extract the active constituents. You should only make Garlic tincture from organically grown *Allium sativum* bulbs, because other forms of Garlic that have been treated with pesticides are not suitable for medicinal use.

The tincture is easy to make and will last for many months if stored in dark glass bottles. For everyday use, you can decant tincture into a small dropper bottle that will fit easily into a purse, briefcase, or pocket.

## TO MAKE A TINCTURE

### STANDARD QUANTITY

8oz (225g) of dried Garlic or 11oz (310g) of fresh Garlic,
4 cups (1 liter) of alcohol and water mixture

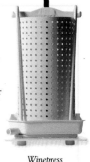

Winepress

1 Roughly chop the Garlic cloves, but leave the skins intact because they will impart important chemicals. Place the cloves in a blender or food processor and cover them with vodka; standard 45% proof is effective, but 70–80% proof is even better.

2 Blend the Garlic and alcohol together. The mixture may be stiff and hard at first, making it difficult for the blades to turn, but persevere. When smooth, pour the mixture into a dark, airtight container; a dark glass jar or preserving jar is ideal.

3 Shake well and then label the jar carefully. Store the jar in a cool place, out of direct sunlight.

4 After two days, measure the contents and add water – just 20% water if you are using standard 45%

proof vodka. However, if you are using 70–80% proof vodka, add 50–60% water to dilute the high alcohol content.

5 When you have added the alcohol and water mixture, cover with a tight-fitting lid and leave the jar for 2–4 weeks, but shake it daily.

6 Strain the mixture through a jelly bag, preferably overnight, or use a home-use winepress (available from drug stores), so that you extract the very last drop. Discard the residual garlic pulp.

7 Pour the liquid into jars, label clearly, and store in a cool, dark place.

Note: It is important always to use utensils that have been cleaned in boiling water – and for the best results, trying adding one or two drops of essential oil, such as lavender, thyme, or tea tree, to the water you use to clean your equipment.

### CAUTION

Do not take this tincture on its own. See Herbal Combinations, pages 47 and 49, for how to use and dosages.

# TINCTURE SYRUP

Garlic tincture is not especially palatable, but when it is combined with honey or maple syrup it becomes much easier to take. Tincture syrup is particularly suitable for young children, especially in the winter, when coughs, colds, and flu germs abound.

## TINCTURES AND THE MOON'S PHASES

Herbalists sometimes time the production of tinctures to coincide with the gravitational waxing and waning of the moon. Start the process when the moon is new, then strain and bottle the tincture at the full moon.

## TO MAKE TINCTURE SYRUP

### STANDARD QUANTITY

Use equal quantities of Garlic tincture and cold-pressed, organic runny honey or maple syrup, plus ½ drop of peppermint essential oil.

1 *In a glass jar, mix equal parts of Garlic tincture and honey or maple syrup. Add extra honey or maple syrup if the Garlic taste is too strong.*

2 *To give the syrup a minty flavor, add the peppermint essential oil. This is popular with children.*

**Recommended dosage**
🌿 *Adults: ½ tsp (2.5ml) 3–6 times daily. Children: over 12 years, ½ tsp (2.5ml) 1–2 times daily; under 12 years, see page 43.*

## REMOVING THE ALCOHOL

You may prefer to avoid the alcohol contained in Garlic tincture, especially if you are diabetic, pregnant, or breastfeeding, or have a history of alcohol or liver problems. If so, add a little boiling water to the dose and let it stand for five minutes. This will cause 98.5% of the alcohol to evaporate. If you want to avoid alcohol completely, replace the alcohol with the same quantity of apple cider vinegar.

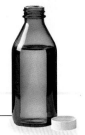

RIGHT **Add peppermint oil to Garlic syrup for a fresh, minty taste.**

# GARLIC CAPSULES

**Kyolic capsules,
tablets, or liquid**

The famous and rightly celebrated natural healer Paavo Airola learned of a novel way of taking Garlic when he toured Japan in the 1970s. He discovered that the Japanese had developed a Garlic supplement known as Kyolic (Kyo-Leopin in Japan, and Leopin in Canada) that "retains all the traditional well-known medicinal and nutritional properties of raw Garlic without Garlic's odor." He describes a special process that involves curing organically grown Garlic in huge vats for 20 months. No heat is used, which ensures that the Garlic retains its healing properties, yet the fermentation process allows its odor to be driven off. Kyolic Garlic is widely available to those people who are embarrassed by the smell.

ABOVE *Odorless Garlic comes in capsules.*

**Recommended dosage**

Adults: 3–4 capsules twice daily or 2–3 tablets 3 times daily. Children: over 12 years, adult dose; under 12 years, see page 43.

**Odorless capsules**

These capsules are also effective but they have not gone through the very gentle and natural fermentation process for removing the odor from the Garlic and, therefore, in my experience, they are not as effective as the Kyolic supplements. If Kyolic capsules are unobtainable, you can certainly substitute other capsules but remember that fresh Garlic, raw or cooked, is always best.

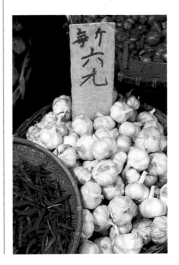

RIGHT *Paavo Airola popularized the use of Kyolic Garlic, which is odor-free.*

# GARLIC IN THE KITCHEN

The best way to benefit from Garlic's healing properties is to cook with it on a regular basis.

Whole bulbs may be cooked with the skin left on. This is traditionally done all over Europe, especially in Greece, Spain, and Italy. Unpeeled cloves or even bulbs are added to stews, casseroles, and other dishes that take a while to cook. Slow cooking allows the goodness and the mouthwatering aroma to seep out gradually.

When Garlic cloves are chopped or crushed, several important sulfur compounds are released. This does not happen when cloves are cooked whole. It is better to chop cloves rather than to crush them, because crushing will destroy most of the active alliin, which is the main active constituent.

A quick way to process a large amount of Garlic is

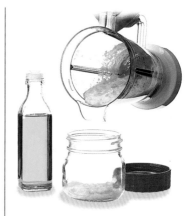

ABOVE *Liquidize fresh garlic with olive oil to make an aromatic paste.*

to liquidize it with olive oil. The resultant paste can then be stored in an airtight glass jar in the refrigerator for use in various dishes during the week. This is convenient because it reduces preparation time and encourages more liberal use of Garlic.

Some health food stores sell Garlic presses, and nonstick presses have recently become available; these extract the juice and many people find them useful. Long before mechanical juice presses were made, Garlic juice and wild thyme were used in combination as a preventative for snakebites.

LEFT *Garlic is delicious sautéed with vegetables before adding to casseroles.*

## GARLIC SOUP

This is a great way to eat Garlic and is very common in the Latin countries of Europe. The quantity of Garlic is a matter of taste, but the more the better. To serve four, try: 1lb (450g) potatoes (unpeeled if organic), 4 cups (1 liter) spring water, 4 medium-size onions (peeled), 3–9 cloves of Garlic (peeled and chopped), and any other culinary herbs desired.

Chop the potatoes into cubes and cook in a pan of boiling water for 10 minutes. Meanwhile chop the onions and fry in a little olive oil. Add the Garlic and any other herbs. Blend the mixture with the spring water and return to the heat. Season to taste.

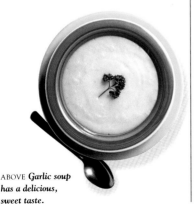

ABOVE **Garlic soup has a delicious, sweet taste.**

### FIGHTER "HOOCH"
Garlic "Hooch" is a mixture of powerful kitchen foods that enhance immunity.

1 Fill a large Mason jar one-quarter full with equal parts of chopped fresh Garlic, chopped fresh white onion (or the hottest onion available), freshly grated ginger root, chopped fresh horseradish if available, and chopped cayenne peppers (again, the hottest available, such as African bird pepper). Top up with organic apple cider vinegar and shake vigorously. (You can liquidize the herbs instead of chopping them.)

2 Filter most of the mixture through cheesecloth or a fine sieve and reserve the liquid. Leave some of the mixture unsieved and use it as a delicious hot relish with food.
Keep in the refrigerator for up to 12 weeks. (If you wish, you can make this formula on the new moon, then strain it on the full moon).

**Recommended dosage**
✤ Adults: 1–2 tbsp (15–30ml) 2 or more times daily. Gargle and swallow.
✤ Children: over 12 years, adult dose; under 12 years, see page 43.

## GARLIC JUICE

To make Garlic juice you will need a juice extractor that is able to process bulky vegetable and fruit matter. Some extractors are combined with a general food processor. When you make the juice, there is no need to peel the bulbs, simply put them whole into the juicer. You will need a great many bulbs to produce a small amount of juice. Try adding one or two cloves of Garlic to other vegetable or fruit juices – it greatly enhances the taste and health benefits. For instance, Garlic juiced with apple makes a superb combination drink to enhance the immune system.

> **CAUTION**
>
> Do not let the extracted juice touch your skin since it will irritate it. Wear plastic gloves while processing Garlic.

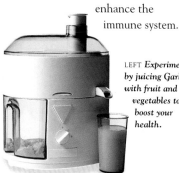

LEFT *Experiment by juicing Garlic with fruit and vegetables to boost your health.*

## GARLIC LEAVES

The leaves of *Allium sativum* have a pleasant taste that is much milder than the bulb. The leaves are very rich in Vitamins A and C and make a healthy addition to stir-fries. Ramsons leaves (from British Wild Garlic – see page 8) are delicious. Collecting bunches of them in the late spring for use in salads and stir-fries is a seasonal joy.

### CASE STUDY: CRADLE CAP

At 5 months old, Mary had persistent cradle cap. It was not unhealthy, but it looked unsightly, and Lucy, her mother, wanted to remove the thick flakes of skin covering her baby's scalp so that the fine skin underneath could "breathe." Lucy had heard an old wives' tale, and decided to try it. The simple remedy had only two ingredients and involved mixing one clove of crudely chopped Garlic with a cup of olive oil and leaving the mixture overnight in a warm place. In the morning Lucy removed the Garlic and massaged the infused olive oil into Mary's scalp. Some of the thick scales came away immediately, and Lucy continued the treatment for just over a week, after which time all the cradle cap had disappeared, revealing the soft skin below.

# GARLIC POWDER

Powdered, dried garlic is very useful for quick and convenient cooking, but always purchase organic powder with a strong aroma. Very versatile, garlic powder can be mixed with olive oil or stirred into a wide variety of dishes. Do not let the powder get damp because, due to its essential oil content, it will clump together and become difficult to use.

Garlic powder is not just beneficial for humans: it is good for the health of many animals too. It has been shown to sweeten the breath of dogs and make their coats shine, for example.

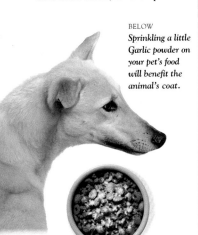

BELOW
*Sprinkling a little Garlic powder on your pet's food will benefit the animal's coat.*

# GARLIC SNUFF

Herbal snuffs are useful for treating nasal congestion and infections. They decongest and drain the sinus cavities, and may even remove infected debris that has been blocking the cavities for many years.

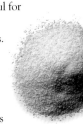

GARLIC SNUFF

### TO MAKE GARLIC SNUFF

**STANDARD QUANTITY**

I part Garlic powder, I part Cayenne powder (optional but excellent), I part Mustard powder

*Mix together all the ingredients and store in an airtight tin.*

**Recommended dosage**

* Adults: 2–4 pinches 3 times daily. Children: over 12 years, adult dose; under 12 years, see page 43.*

*Place a minute amount on the back of your hand and close one nostril. Snort up the snuff into the open nostril. To keep the snuff in the back of the nasal cavity, hold the head back for as long as possible. Repeat on the other side.*

---

#### CAUTION

Consult a doctor or herbalist before taking snuff. Do not take it if you have asthma.

# Preparations for external use

A WIDE RANGE OF CONDITIONS *can be treated when Garlic is applied topically, but care must be taken that its effect is well buffered by applying it with other substances, so that the skin is not irritated in the process.*

GARLIC
OINTMENT

## GARLIC OINTMENT

An ointment containing Garlic is useful for bites, cuts, and wounds, although it is not appropriate for those who mind the smell. It can also make a very safe cure-all ointment for animals (with the permission of your vet) and I have used it to treat cuts on horses, dogs, and cats.

### TO MAKE AN OINTMENT

#### STANDARD QUANTITY

1½ cups (350ml) of olive oil, 8oz (225g) dried, powdered Garlic, ¼oz (5g) beeswax

1 Mix the olive oil and Garlic together and put in a heatproof, covered container. Place in the oven at 104°F (40°C) for an hour, or stand it in the sun or a warm spot for a week. Stir with a fork.

2 Leave for another week to macerate. Reheat, then strain by passing through a large colander lined with a piece of cheesecloth, or by using a jelly bag.

3 Melt the beeswax at a very low temperature and add the herbal olive oil mixture. Have sterilized, dark glass jars ready and put a little of the liquid into one of them to check the consistency; it should be similar to runny honey when pouring into the jar. Let it set; this should take about two minutes in the refrigerator. When the mixture solidifies to the consistency of a cold cream, put it into the jars.

## GARLIC COMPRESS

A compress is a piece of cloth soaked in Garlic decoction and applied to the affected part. Garlic's powerful chemicals travel swiftly around the body getting to work immediately at the site of the problem. Apply a compress to the nose or chest for respiratory infections. It is wise to take Garlic internally as well as externally for best results.

### TO MAKE A COMPRESS

**STANDARD QUANTITY**

1 Garlic bulb, 3 cups (750ml) spring water

1 *Using a darning needle, pierce a Garlic bulb all over to make many little holes. This ensures that the active ingredients will be released into the water. Alternatively, peel the cloves and use them together with the skins.*

2 *Place the bulb, or the cloves and skins, with the spring water in a saucepan or a double boiler. Simmer the decoction on a very low heat for about 20–30 minutes. During this time the liquid will reduce down by about one-third.*

3 *Remove the decoction from the heat, and let it cool thoroughly.*

4 *When the decoction is cool, strain it through a plastic or stainless steel sieve into a pitcher.*

5 *Soak a soft, clean cloth (cheesecloth is ideal) in the cooled decoction and wring out the excess liquid.*

6 *Place the compress on the affected area and leave it in position for no longer than five minutes. Inhale the Garlic aroma deeply for best results. This compress can be very useful for the lungs if there is a stubborn infection or congestion.*

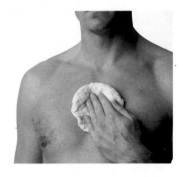

## DR. CHRISTOPHER'S EAR DROPS

This formula is ideal for problems ranging from ear infections to Ménière's disease. It was used for more than 50 years with great success by Dr. John Christopher (1909–82).

### TO MAKE DR. CHRISTOPHER'S EAR DROPS

**STANDARD QUANTITY**

2 parts Vervain tincture, 2 parts Blue Cohosh tincture, 2 parts Black Cohosh tincture, 2 parts Skullcap tincture, ½ part Lobelia seed tincture, 2–4 parts Garlic and Mullein oil (see right)

*Combine the tinctures. Mix one part of the combined tinctures with 2–4 parts of Garlic and Mullein Herbal Oil (see right). Pour into a sterilized, dark glass dropper bottle.*

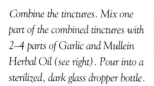

### Recommended dosage

🦴 *Adults: 6–8 gently warmed drops **in both ears** once a night, and plug with absorbent cotton. In the morning, flush ears with ¼ part gently warmed water and ¼ part cider vinegar. Children: over 12 years, adult dose, 7–12 years and over, half adult dose; 3–7 years, 2–3 drops; babies: 1 drop each ear.*

### TO MAKE GARLIC AND MULLEIN HERBAL OIL

**STANDARD QUANTITY**

Use 10 Garlic cloves, 1 cup (250 ml) extra virgin olive oil, 1 tbsp (15ml) powdered dried Mullein

1 *Purée the Garlic and olive oil in a blender. Place in a covered, ovenproof container in an oven at 104°F (40°C) for half a day.*

2 *Remove from the oven, add the Mullein, and mix well. Allow to macerate for 3 days, then strain, bottle and label ready for use.*

*Note: You can vary the amount of Garlic and Mullein oil you add to the ear drops – reduce the quantity for those who are sensitive to Garlic's smell.*

RIGHT **Mullein is a remedy for ear infections.**

---

CAUTION

Consult a doctor for acute or persistent earache, particularly in children under 12.

---

NOTE

Lobelia is only available from qualified herbalists. Omit the Lobelia when making the ear drops, or ask a herbalist for the formula.

# WHOLE GARLIC SUPPOSITORIES AND GARLIC DOUCHES

Treating vaginal infection with Garlic has been practiced for many centuries. It is a very useful home remedy to know about and women still use it frequently. The antiseptic properties of Garlic are very powerful. The herb can help to treat any condition from candida (thrush) to leucorrhea.

Choose a very large, single clove of Garlic, at least half the size of your thumb. It is important to use a very large clove because small cloves can get lost in the vagina. Place in the vagina. Replace every few hours, or simply use one a day for two hours. You can repeat this procedure over a span of 3–7 days.

Consult a doctor or a herbalist if the condition does not clear up within one week.

On no account pierce the skin of the peeled Garlic clove if you find you are very sensitive – leave the clove's skin covering intact. However, if you find you are not too sensitive, make a tiny sharp piercing in one place so that more of the desirable qualities seep out.

Alternatively, break open a Garlic capsule and apply 2 drops of oil to a tampon. You can leave it in place for a maximum of 1 hour. You can also use douches to support the treatment.

## TO MAKE A VAGINAL DOUCHE

### STANDARD QUANTITY

1 medium-size clove of Garlic,
3 cups (750ml) water, 4 tbsp (60ml)
apple cider vinegar, juice
of 1 organic lemon or lime

*Combine all the ingredients in a food processor, then strain through a colander or sieve lined with cheesecloth. Use as normal for a douche, following the*

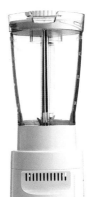

*instructions that come with a douche kit. (Douche kits are available from some health food and nutrition stores as well as pharmacies.)*

LEFT **Blend Garlic to make a natural treatment for thrush.**

## GARLIC POULTICES

A poultice is a healing remedy for wounds or cuts where disinfecting is important. Garlic is a prime anti-infection herb and is therefore ideal in poultice formulas. Sometimes poultices are required to help tissue grow back, or to draw out impurities and poisons.

### TO MAKE A POULTICE TO AID HEALING

**STANDARD QUANTITY**

6 parts Slippery Elm powder, 3 parts Comfrey root powder, 1 part Garlic powder, 2 tbsp Aloe Vera juice, and enough olive oil or St. John's Wort oil to make a paste

1 *Mix together the dry ingredients and moisten into a claylike consistency using equal parts of Aloe Vera juice with either olive oil or St. John's Wort oil.*

2 *Smear carefully onto the clean wound.*

3 *Once or twice a day apply more poultice. Only ever put more poultices on the wound; never remove the previous application. The poultice should only be removed when the wound has healed. When showering or bathing, cover the affected area with plastic wrap to keep it dry.*

### TO MAKE A POULTICE TO DRAW OUT IMPURITIES

**STANDARD QUANTITY**

6 parts Slippery Elm powder, 2 parts Charcoal powder, 1 part Garlic powder, 2 tbsp Aloe Vera juice, and enough olive oil or St. John's Wort oil to make a paste

1 *Mix together the dry ingredients and moisten into a claylike consistency using equal parts of Aloe Vera juice with either olive oil or St. John's Wort oil.*

2 *Apply to the wound and cover with a clean piece of gauze.*

3 *Change dressings frequently, at least every morning and night. This is necessary to clear the impurities that the poultice draws out. When bathing, cover the affected area with plastic wrap to keep it dry.*

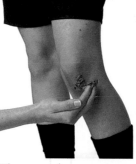

ABOVE
**A herbal poultice will soon heal minor cuts.**

# OTHER APPLICATIONS

## Garlic paste

This is a very old remedy used by generations of herbalists and households from the 1920s onward. It has never been completely out of favor, although its popularity has dwindled. The famous herbalist Dr. John Christopher used it a great deal.

Fresh Garlic paste is smeared onto the soles of feet and left for several hours, or overnight. Garlic is an antiseptic herb. Used in this way it can treat fever and some bronchial and respiratory disorders, particularly if they are stubborn and long-lasting.

To make the paste, peel 12 Garlic cloves and place them in a blender with enough Vaseline (petroleum jelly) to make the blades turn.

You should coat the feet up to the ankles with olive oil, to prevent any of the Garlic from making direct contact with the skin of the feet or ankles. Then divide the resulting Garlic paste in two and, using your hands protected by plastic gloves, smear a deep layer of the paste onto the soles of the feet. If the Garlic paste doesn't contain enough Vaseline, it will easily burn the tender skin on the soles of the feet, which is painful. If you experience hot, burning, or tingling sensations at any time, remove the paste, and apply Aloe Vera gel.

The Garlic paste is best applied for 1–2 hours during the day, but seasoned users can keep it on overnight. It may be smelled on the breath 20 minutes after the paste is applied, showing how quickly it can enter and travel around the body.

ABOVE **Eventually the whole of the feet, including the toes, are covered with plastic wrap.**

## To use

❋ Coat the feet up to the ankles in olive oil.

❦ Smear the soles of the feet with Garlic paste.

❋ Cover the entire foot up to the ankles with plastic wrap, ensuring that the toes are also covered.

❋ Cover all with old socks.

❋ Sit for 1–2 hours with your feet raised up; do not walk around.

People who have used the paste before can do this overnight.

# Natural medicine for everyone

GARLIC IS A SAFE HERBAL REMEDY *that is usually ideal for everyone. However, if you find that it upsets you, follow your body's warning signs and omit it from your diet.*

## PREGNANCY

Garlic can be enjoyed safely throughout pregnancy. It promotes good health in general, and in particular it boosts the digestive and immune systems. It is sometimes not advisable to prescribe antibiotics for pregnant women, and in these cases Garlic is a natural antibiotic alternative.

Research has shown that Garlic has a growth-promoting effect on the cells of the placenta, an action that can help prevent or lessen the effect of some pregnancy complications. By improving the functioning of the placenta, which nourishes the fetus, Garlic is believed to help prevent low birthweight in babies.

Smoking is a cause of low birthweight, so if you cannot give up smoking, adding Garlic to your diet may alleviate some of the effects.

Garlic can also reduce other placental problems, such as pre-eclampsia (raised blood pressure and protein in the urine). Some of Garlic's effectiveness appears to be due to the reduction in activity of key enzymes that are produced in abnormal pregnancies.

LEFT *Garlic is an excellent tonic food for pregnant women.*

## CHILDREN

If all children eat Garlic from an early age, they will accept it as a normal part of life, as children do in southern Europe. Garlic keeps children in good health. In particular it is a natural antibiotic and will make them less prone to coughs, colds, flu, and other common infections. This is of great importance now that doctors are reluctant to prescribe antibiotics. Cooking with Garlic is safe for children of all ages, but consult a herbal practitioner before giving children under 12 medicinal doses of Garlic.

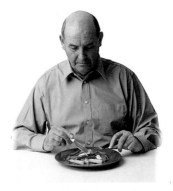

ABOVE **Adding Garlic to meals is a ticket to a long and healthy old age.**

BELOW **Garlic helps children stay healthy.**

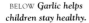

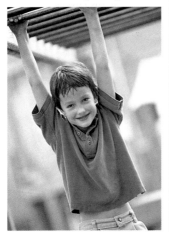

## ELDERLY PEOPLE

The immune, circulatory, and digestive systems all become weakened with age. The elderly are advised to use Garlic both in cooking and medicinally, to help slow down or reverse this effect. Unlike children, the elderly are likely to have antibiotics prescribed for them by doctors, but increasingly antibiotics are not working in the same way as in the past, now that antibiotic-resistant bacteria are emerging. Garlic has a great role to play in preventing the need for such antibiotics. It is also an excellent remedy for heart health, and can help to reduce blood pressure and atherosclerosis.

# Herbal combinations

GARLIC IS A PROFOUND HEALER *in its own right but it can be combined with other herbs, either to buffer its sometimes "piercing" effect or to produce a wider spectrum of actions.*

## CLEANSING AND DETOXIFYING THE COLON

This formula is useful to help relieve symptoms of a malfunctioning colon, such as constipation, wind, and cramps. It also helps to reduce overgrowth of candida, a fungus that is naturally present in the gut. If candida multiplies too quickly, it can cause bloating, wind, and constipation alternating with diarrhea. The formula provokes the bowel to work, and will relieve wind or cramp. Over a period of time the formula will strengthen the walls of the small intestine, and destroy

ABOVE **Aloe Vera** *leaves contain laxative properties.*

candida and other fungal, parasitic, and viral invasions. Garlic is antiseptic and antifungal, while Senna, Aloe, Cascara, and Barberry all have a laxative effect. Ginger, Peppermint, and Fennel ease any wind or cramp.

**Formula** 2 parts Aloe Vera leaf powder, 1 part Senna leaves and pods powder, ½ or 1 part (depending on strength of formula desired) Cascara Sagrada powder, 1 part Barberry root bark powder, 1 part Ginger, Peppermint or Fennel seed powder, 1 part organic Garlic powder, 1 part organic hot Cayenne powder.

**To make** Mix the powders in a
flat dish or saucer, then scoop
them into 00-size vegetarian or
gelatin capsules and join the
halves together. Each capsule will
take about 200–250mg of powder.
Store the capsules in a sterilized,
dark glass, labeled jar.

**Dosage** Adults: take 1 capsule
on the first night and ensuing
nights, and then increase the
dose by an extra capsule per
night until a suitable personal
dose is found.

Children: over 12 years, adult
dose; under 12 years, see page 43.

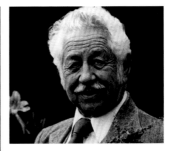

ABOVE *Dr. Christopher treated
soldiers during World War II
with herbal remedies.*

---

CAUTION

Do not take this colon formula if you are
pregnant, breastfeeding, or suffering from
hemorrhoids, colitis, or kidney disease.

---

## DR. CHRISTOPHER'S ANTIPLAGUE FORMULA

Dr. Christopher's antiplague
formula takes its name from its
ability to relieve outbreaks of
rapid infection. It can treat
influenza, salmonella, and other
gastrointestinal problems causing
diarrhea and vomiting. The
formula is as relevant today as it
was in Dr. Christopher's lifetime.

Dr. Christopher's 50 years of
practice included treating soldiers
with herbs during World War II,
where quick-spreading infections
were all too familiar.

The herbs in the formula are
antiseptic and antimicrobial.
They also keep the immune,
circulatory, and lymph systems
working at optimum levels, while
nourishing and calming the
nervous system.

---

CAUTION

Dr. Christopher's antiplague formula
contains very powerful herbs. Do not take
it if you have bowel disorders such as colitis
or Irritable Bowel Syndrome (IBS) except
under the supervision of a qualified herbal
practitioner. Do not take for more than
one week except on the advice of a
herbal practitioner.

---

**Formula** 1 part each of the following tinctures: Black Walnut, Wormwood herb pods, Marshmallow leaves, Oak bark, Lobelia leaf, Mullein leaf, Skullcap leaf, and Uva Ursi leaves, plus 2 parts Gravel root tincture or decoction, 2 parts Burdock root tincture, 2 parts fresh organic Garlic juice, 5 parts organic, unfiltered, cold-pressed honey, 5 parts vegetable glycerin, and 8 parts apple cider vinegar.

**To make** Juice the Garlic (see page 34) using fresh organic cloves. Make the tinctures (see page 29) or buy them from herbal stores. Mix the tinctures together, then add the Garlic juice, honey, vegetable glycerin, and cider vinegar. Pour the formula into a sterilized, dark glass bottle that is clearly labeled. Only make as much as you need, and store for no longer than 3–4 days in the refrigerator; the formula can

last longer, but works better when fresh. Alternatively, mix the tinctures and other ingredients except the Garlic juice up to 1–2 years in advance. The Garlic juice can be made and added to the formula at the last moment on the day it is required.

**Dosage** Adults: 1 tsp (5ml) 3–5 times daily with water for as long as the symptoms persist. More doses will do no harm and for severe situations you can take up to 1 tbsp (15ml) every half hour. You can also take 1–2 tsp (5–10ml) once during the night if desired. Take doses with a little food if your stomach is sensitive to Garlic; this will help to protect the lining of the stomach.

Children: over 12 years, adult dose; under 12 years, see page 43.

**CAUTION**

Do not take Dr. Christopher's formula if you are pregnant.

**NOTE**

Lobelia is only available from qualified herbalists. Omit the Lobelia when making the drops, or ask a herbalist for the formula.

RIGHT
*Skullcap leaves and flowers.*

# DIABETES

Garlic helps to treat diabetes by reducing the amount of sugar in the blood and stimulating the pancreas to produce more insulin. Garlic's benefits for the circulation and immune system also help those with diabetes, even when the disease is so severe that the circulation has become impaired.

As well as containing Garlic, this remedy features Fenugreek and Burdock, both of which are renowned for balancing blood-sugar levels, and Astragalus and Siberian Ginseng, which are herbs that help improve the body's energy levels. This formula is also a tonic for the endocrine system, of which the pancreas is a part.

The formula can be further reinforced by adding additional herbs that support the endocrine system. For example, you can try adding Agnus Castus (which is suitable for both men and women), or Saw Palmetto (generally suitable for men only).

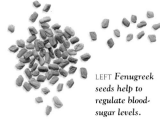

LEFT *Fenugreek seeds help to regulate blood-sugar levels.*

**Formula** Equal parts of Garlic tincture, Fenugreek seed tincture, Burdock root tincture, Juniper berry tincture, Siberian Ginseng tincture, Astragalus tincture. Optional: 1 part Agnus Castus tincture (suitable for both sexes) or Saw Palmetto tincture (suitable for men only). You can also add ¼ part Stevia tincture for sweetness and support for the pancreas.

**To make** Mix the tinctures together and store in a sterilized, dark glass, labeled bottle.

**Dosage** Adults: 1 tsp (5ml) 4–6 times daily with water.

Children: over 12 years, adult dose; under 12 years, see page 43.

ABOVE *Siberian Ginseng root is an ancient Chinese energy herb.*

### CAUTION

Consult your doctor before taking this formula for diabetes.

## LIVER FLUSH

This formula improves liver function. It helps to treat jaundice, hepatitis C, constant nausea and sickness, chronic indigestion, and premenstrual syndrome. This gentle liver flush, which should be used for 1–2 days, contains lemon juice, a citrus acid that becomes alkaline in the stomach and cleanses the digestive tract. It also emulsifies the olive oil and creates a fresh, palatable flavor. Olive oil has a cleansing action, and Ginger is a well-known digestive stimulant. Seek professional help before starting a cleanse because the powerful effects need monitoring.

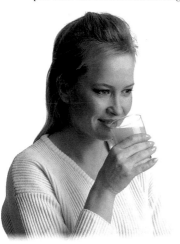

**Formula** 1–2 freshly squeezed lemons, ¾ cup (200ml) freshly squeezed (or carton) apple juice, ¾ cup (200ml) spring water, 1 crushed clove of fresh Garlic, 1 tbsp (15 ml) extra virgin olive oil, and ¼in (5mm) peeled, chopped fresh Ginger root. Note: omit the Ginger if your liver feels hot and inflamed.

**To make** Purée all the ingredients in a blender until smooth.

**Dosage** Adults: The aim is to drink the whole dose first thing in the morning on an empty stomach for up to 2 consecutive mornings. Start with a small quantity and build up gradually. If you have headaches and feel "unwell," do not repeat for a week. Follow with organic apple juice if desired, and 15 minutes later drink a cup of hot Peppermint tea (preferably made with fresh leaves), or Dandelion coffee flavored with Cinnamon sticks, Cardamom seed, grated Ginger, or a little Licorice.

Children: seek professional herbal or medical advice before beginning this cleanse.

LEFT *Garlic, lemon, and apple juice flush out toxins and restore the liver to full health.*

**Side-effects** When the liver clears out, headaches, rashes, and other side-effects occur, which are a sign that the detoxification process is under way. Emotional reactions can also arise, and you may feel depressed or angry. Stop if symptoms are intolerable but, if bearable, repeat the next morning. Drink lots of water and eat as normal all day (wholesome, healthy food, rich in vegetables or fruits, raw and cooked). Do not fast during the cleanse because the effects will be too intense.

## HIGH BLOOD PRESSURE FORMULA

High blood pressure may be caused by extreme stress, but often cholesterol levels may be too high, kidneys sluggish, and the blood too thick. If this is the case, this formula is ideal. Garlic and Ginkgo improve circulation and reduce blood cholesterol levels, which otherwise build up on coronary artery walls, pushing up blood pressure. Uva Ursi and Dandelion have a diuretic effect and reduce the overall volume of fluid in the body, which helps lower blood pressure. Hawthorn relaxes and dilates the coronary

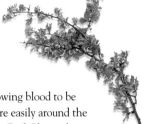

RIGHT
*Hawthorn has been proven to help lower blood pressure.*

arteries, allowing blood to be pumped more easily around the body. Finally, Red Clover thins and detoxifies the blood.

**Formula** Equal parts of tinctures of Hawthorn leaf, berry, and flower, Red Clover flower, Ginkgo leaf, Uva Ursi leaf, Dandelion root, Garlic clove (or freshly juiced Garlic).

**To make** Mix the ingredients and store in sterilized, dark glass, labeled bottles. If using Garlic juice, add just before taking.

**Dosage** Adults: 1 tsp (5ml) 3–4 times daily. In addition, consume 3 raw Garlic cloves a day or take 2 Garlic capsules (see page 31) 3 times a day. Also, drink 4 cups (1 liter) of spring water a day to flush out the kidneys. Children: seek professional herbal or medical advice.

---

### CAUTION

Always seek professional advice for high blood pressure.

---

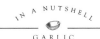

---

# Conditions chart

THIS CHART IS A GUIDE to some of the ailments that Garlic can treat, but it is not intended to replace other forms of treatment. Always consult your doctor or another qualified medical practitioner before embarking on a course of treatment.

| NAME | INTERNAL USE | EXTERNAL USE |
| --- | --- | --- |
| **ABSCESS** | Tincture or capsule, or in food | Ointment or poultice |
| **ACNE** | Tincture or capsule, or in food | Ointment or poultice |
| **ARTHRITIS** | Tincture or capsule, or in food | Ointment |
| **ASTHMA** | Tincture or capsule, or in food | Garlic paste |
| **ATHLETE'S FOOT** | Tincture or capsule, or in food | Ointment or Garlic paste |
| **BOILS** | Tincture or capsule, or in food | Poultice |
| **BRONCHITIS** | Tincture or capsule, or in food | Garlic paste |
| **CIRCULATION** | Tincture or capsule, or in food | |
| **COLDS** | Tincture or capsule, or in food | |
| **DIABETES** | Tincture or capsule, or in food | |

| NAME | INTERNAL USE | EXTERNAL USE |
|---|---|---|
| **EARACHE** | Tincture or capsule, or in food | Ear drops |
| **ECZEMA** | Tincture or capsule, or in food | |
| **FLATULENCE** | Tincture or capsule, or in food | |
| **FLU** | Tincture or capsule, or in food | Garlic paste |
| **HEPATITIS** | Tincture or capsule, or in food | |
| **HIGH BLOOD PRESSURE** | Tincture or capsule, or in food | |
| **LEUCORRHEA** | Tincture or capsule, or in food | |
| **MALARIA** | Tincture or capsule, or in food | |
| **MASTITIS** | Tincture or capsule, or in food | |
| **PARASITES** | Tincture or capsule, or in food | |
| **PLEURISY** | Tincture or capsule, or in food | |
| **PNEUMONIA** | Tincture or capsule, or in food | |
| **PREGNANCY COMPLAINTS** | Tincture or capsule, or in food | |
| **SORES** | Tincture or capsule, or in food | Ointment and poultice |
| **SORE THROAT** | Tincture or capsule, or in food | |
| **TONSILLITIS** | Tincture or capsule, or in food | |
| **ULCERS** | Tincture or capsule, or in food | |
| **WHOOPING COUGH** | Tincture or capsule, or in food | |

# How Garlic works

GARLIC HAS NEARLY *20 major chemical actions in the body, all with profound effects. To date, 33 sulfur compounds have been found in Garlic, the largest quantity so far discovered in a plant. Each of these have different roles. Among sulfur's many attributes is its ability to break down cholesterol – good news given the high-fat diets that so many people consume nowadays.*

Garlic has the following chemical properties and other components:

❋ Alliin: A sulfur that contains an amino acid from which allicin is made. Alliin can kill a wide spectrum of unfavorable microbes and bacteria.

❋ Allicin: Responsible for Garlic's odor, it contributes to the plant's effectiveness as an antibacterial agent. Allicin also has anti-inflammatory abilities, which makes it useful for many autoimmune diseases. Allicin is activated only when the cloves are cut or crushed (it eventually becomes diallyldisulfide oxide, in a series of natural reactions). However, it is best not to crush Garlic (see page 32).

❋ Allithiamine: Formed when vitamin B$_1$, or thiamine, in Garlic reacts with alliin. Vitamin B$_1$ naturally contains sulfur.

❋ Biotin: another B vitamin found in Garlic, which also contains sulfur. Vitamin B$_1$ and

LEFT **Many cooks crush Garlic, but it is better to chop it.**

biotin both nourish the nervous system and brain. This happens partly because the sulfur they contain can force lecithin (needed for brain chemistry) into the brain and nervous system. They also help prevent cholesterol from depositing in the arteries.

✽ Essential oil: Lowers cholesterol and lipid (fat) levels in the blood. It has an extremely strong, long-lasting odor, which is not necessarily a bad thing because the odor also heals the body.

✽ Selenium: A useful sulfur-type trace mineral that has antioxidant properties. Selenium may help inhibit cancer formation. It also helps prevent heavy metals from damaging the body.

✽ Germanium: A trace mineral with a number of positive attributes, one being that it is a powerful antioxidant.

✽ Gurwitch rays: Emitted by Garlic, these are an unusual type of ultraviolet radiation called Mitogenic Radiation. The rays have stimulating growth capabilities and can rejuvenate the whole body (see page 55).

## CASE STUDY: GALLBLADDER

Mark, an engineer in his 40s, suffered from extremely bad heartburn that left him in pain for hours at a time. It was particularly bad at night, preventing him from sleeping. Mark had had his gallbladder removed two years previously, and at the time his herbal practitioner had warned that his liver and stomach would need special care because they would be taking over some of the work that his gallbladder had been doing.

One night, Mark happened to eat a pasta dish that contained ample quantities of Garlic. That evening his heartburn did not appear. He told his herbalist, who suggested that he continued to eat plenty of Garlic and explained that the herb can help the digestive system metabolize fats. Mark started using Garlic liberally in cooking and his heartburn vanished. To date, it has not returned.

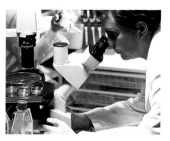

ABOVE *Scientists around the world are researching Garlic's properties.*

## MAIN EFFECTS

Garlic has the following effects:

🗦 Thins the blood, increases the circulation, and reduces blood-platelet clumping and stickiness.

🗦 Destroys fungi, viruses, bacteria, and parasites.

🗦 Normalizes blood pressure, whether high or low.

🗦 Helps lower high cholesterol and triglyceride levels.

🗦 Balances high and low blood-sugar levels.

🗦 Helps neutralize and remove heavy metals from the body.

🗦 Assists the immune system in many ways, partly by calming and repairing the entire system.

🗦 Treats autoimmune diseases, such as rheumatoid arthritis, where there is excessive inflammation of an imbalanced immune system.

🗦 Antioxidant action helps to reduce the degeneration that is a feature of many chronic diseases and slows down the aging process.

## RESEARCH

Louis Pasteur was one of the first people to discover Garlic's remarkable properties – he found that it had a very similar antibiotic effect to penicillin. Currently, scientists are researching Garlic's antibacterial and antifungal qualities and investigating it as a remedy for diabetes, heart disease, stroke, and cancer. Japanese research, for example, shows that Garlic is rich in germanium, a trace mineral that can help treat and prevent low blood sugar, diabetes, and cancer. Researchers in the United States and in Oxford, United

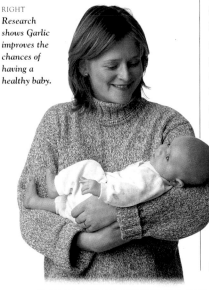

RIGHT
*Research shows Garlic improves the chances of having a healthy baby.*

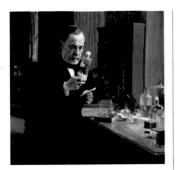

ABOVE *Louis Pasteur (1822–1895) discovered Garlic's antibiotic effects.*

Kingdom, have found that Garlic supplements help to reduce high blood cholesterol levels. In trials a reduction in total cholesterol of 12 percent was achieved after four weeks. Garlic also significantly lowered triglycerides (potentially harmful blood fats).

Research by Dr. Paavo Airola, in Kerala, India, showed that Garlic reduced lipid (fat) levels in the blood and in the liver. Dr. Airola also reported on clinical trials on 114 patients in Germany that proved Garlic can reduce high blood pressure and arteriosclerosis.

Garlic also reduces blood-sugar levels. In a German study there was an 11 percent reduction in the blood-sugar levels of people taking Garlic. Research in the United States showed that Garlic releases 15 different kinds of antioxidant chemicals. According to research, the plant also improves male fertility and libido levels, and can help to strengthen or induce an erection.

Taking Garlic during pregnancy may cut the risk of preeclampsia (see page 57). Research at the Chelsea & Westminster Hospital in London, United Kingdom, also found that if pregnant women regularly ate Garlic, they were less likely to have a low-birthweight baby.

A Russian electrobiologist, Professor Gurwitch, discovered that Garlic emits a type of ultraviolet radiation called Mitogenic Radiations. Now referred to as Gurwitch rays, they have a cell-stimulating growth capability and a generalized rejuvenating effect on the body.

Finally, Bernard Jensen at the University of California, Los Angeles, found that Garlic extract retarded the growth of skin cancer cells.

# Glossary

**AMINO ACIDS**
Chemically simple substances of which proteins are composed.

**ANEMIA**
A condition in which there is too little hemoglobin, the oxygen-carrying pigment of red blood cells.

**ANTHRAX**
An infectious disease that is caused by Bacillus anthracis, a rod-shaped bacterium. This disease attacks the skin and lungs and can be transmitted from farm animals to humans by contact with animal hair.

**ANTIBIOTIC**
Fights bacterial infections.

**ANTI-INFLAMMATORY**
Reduces inflammation.

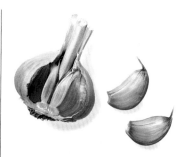

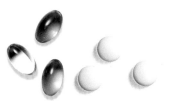

**ANTIMICROBIAL**
Destroys or inhibits the growth of microorganisms.

**ANTIOXIDANTS**
Substances found in a wide range of fruit and vegetables that prevent oxidation and breakdown of body tissues.

**DIURETIC**
Promotes urination.

**ENDAMEBA HISTOLYTICA**
Bacteria that causes amebic dysentery. It is contracted from contaminated water or food.

**ENDOCRINE GLAND**
A gland that releases a hormone

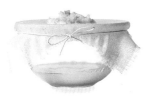

directly into the bloodstream to act on other parts of the body.

### ENDOCRINE SYSTEM

A collection of glands that produce hormones. It includes the pituitary, thyroid, parathyroid, adrenal, and pineal glands.

### FATTY ACIDS

Substances found in foods that contain fats and oils.

### FLAVONOIDS

Compounds in plants responsible for a wide range of actions, including

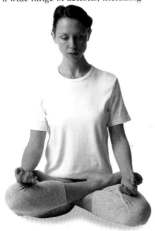

reducing inflammation and improving the circulation.

### GIARDIA LAMBLIA

A microscopic parasite that lives in the intestine. It can cause chronic diarrhea and malnutrition because of malabsorption of food.

### IMMUNE SYSTEM

A collection of specialized cells and proteins in the body that fend off foreign bodies, such as fungi, viruses, and bacteria.

### LEUCORRHEA

Excessive vaginal discharge.

### PREECLAMPSIA

A serious condition that can occur in the second half of pregnancy. Symptoms include high blood pressure and protein in the urine.

### STEROL

A steroid alcohol. Sterols found in plants are known as phytosterols.

### SULFUR

Component of many vitamins and proteins, especially muscle proteins. In plants it is essential for growth.

### TUBERCULOSIS

A disease that affects the lungs.

# Further reading

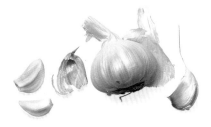

BRITISH HERBAL PHARMACOPOEIA
1996 (British Herbal Medical
Association, 1996)

COMPLETE GARLIC HANDBOOK,
*Peter Josling* (Carnell plc, 1996)

ENCYCLOPAEDIA OF MEDICINAL
PLANTS, *Andrew Chevallier* (Dorling
Kindersley, 1996)

ESSENTIAL SCIENCE CHEMISTRY,
*Freemantle & Tidy* (Oxford
University Press, 1983)

FIELD GUIDE TO WILD FLOWERS,
*Roger Peterson & Margaret McKenny*
(Houghton Mifflin Company, 1968)

GARLIC'S HEALING POWERS,
*Bernard Jensen* (Bernard Jensen
Publisher, 1992)

THE HERBAL FOR MOTHER AND
CHILD, *Anne McIntyre*
(Element, 1992)

HOME HERBAL, *Penelope Ody*
(Dorling Kindersley, 1995)

MANUAL OF CONVENTIONAL
MEDICINE FOR ALTERNATIVE
PRACTITIONERS, *Stephen Gascoigne*
(Jigame Press, 1993)

MIRACLE OF GARLIC, *Paavo Airola*
(Health Plus, 1996)

A MODERN HERBAL, *Mrs. M. Grieve*
(Tiger Books, 1992)

SCHOOL OF NATURAL HEALING,
*Dr. Christopher* (Christopher
Publications, 1976)

TEXTBOOK OF ADVANCED
HERBOLOGY, *Terry Willard* (Wild
Rose College of Natural Healing,
1992)

THORSON'S GUIDE TO MEDICAL
HERBALISM, *David Hoffman*
(Thorsons, 1991)

# Useful addresses

ASSOCIATIONS AND SOCIETIES

**British Herbal Medicine
Association (B.H.M.A)**
Sun House, Church Street, Stroud,
Glos. GL5 1JL, UK
Tel: 011 44 1453–751389
Fax: 011 44 1453–751402
Works with the Medicine Control
Agency to promote high standards of
quality and safety of herbal medicine

**Herb Society**
Deddington Hill Farm,
Warmington, Banbury,
Oxon OX17 1XB, UK
Tel: 011 44 1295–692000
Fax: 011 44 1295–692004
Educational charity that disseminates
information about herbs and
organizes workshops

**The Wild Plant Conservation
Charity**
The Natural History Museum,
Cromwell Road,
London SW7 5BD, UK
Tel: 011 44 171–938 9123
Registered charity to save British
wild plants

SUPPLIERS IN THE UK

**Baldwin & Company**
171–173 Walworth Road,
London SE17 1RW, UK
Tel: 011 44 171–703 5550
Herbs, storage bottles, jars, and
containers available

**Hambleden Herbs**
Court Farm, Milverton,
Somerset TA4 1NF, UK
Tel: 011 44 1823–401205
Organic herbs by mail order

**Herbs, Hands, Healing**
The Cabins, Station Warehouse,
Station Road, Pulham Market,
Norfolk IP21 4XF, UK
Tel: 011 44 1379–608007
Tel/fax: 011 44 1379–608201
Organic herbal formulas &
Superfood; mail order; free brochure

SUPPLIERS/SCHOOLS IN THE USA

**American Botanical Pharmacy**
PO Box 3027, Santa Monica,
CA 90408, USA
Tel/fax: 1310 453–1987
Manufacturer and distributor of
herbal products; runs training courses

**Blessed Herbs**
109 Barre Plains Road,
Oakham,
MA 01068, USA
Tel: 1800 489–4372
Dried bulk herbs are available by
mail order in order to make your
own preparations

**United Plant Savers**
PO Box 420,
E. Barre,
VT 05649, USA
Aims to preserve wild Native
American medicinal plants

*Other Healing Herb Books
in the Nutshell Series*

❧

ECHINACEA
*ECHINACEA ANGUSTIFOLIA
ECHINACEA PURPUREA*

❧

GINKGO
*GINKGO BILOBA*

❧

GINSENG
*ELEUTHEROCOCCUS SENTICOSUS*

❧

HAWTHORN
*CRATAEGUS MONOGYNA*

❧

MARIGOLD
*CALENDULA OFFICINALIS*

❧

ST. JOHN'S WORT
*HYPERICUM PERFORATUM*

❧

SAW PALMETTO
*SERENOA SERRULATA*